FROM THE
PLANE
TO THE
PLANET

FROM THE
PLANE
TO THE
PLANET

MY PLANT-BASED JOURNEY

PATRICIA A. MORGAN

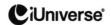

FROM THE PLANE TO THE PLANET
MY PLANT-BASED JOURNEY

You should not undertake any diet/exercise regimen recommended in this book before consulting your personal physician. Neither the author nor the publisher shall be responsible or liable for any loss or damage allegedly arising as a consequence of your use or application of any information or suggestions contained in this book.

iUniverse books may be ordered through booksellers or by contacting:

iUniverse
1663 Liberty Drive
Bloomington, IN 47403
www.iuniverse.com
844-349-9409

Because of the dynamic nature of the Internet, any web addresses or links contained in this book may have changed since publication and may no longer be valid. The views expressed in this work are solely those of the author and do not necessarily reflect the views of the publisher, and the publisher hereby disclaims any responsibility for them.

Any people depicted in stock imagery provided by Getty Images are models, and such images are being used for illustrative purposes only. Certain stock imagery © Getty Images.

ISBN: 978-1-6632-5182-4 (sc)
ISBN: 978-1-6632-5189-3 (e)

Library of Congress Control Number: 2023905548

Print information available on the last page.

iUniverse rev. date: 05/15/2023

To everyone who will or has already
decided to honor their bodies to be
in alignment with the planet:
may you find great joy and
contentment as a gem that
most will never find

JOB OFFER

After months of looking for work, I finally got a job offer to work in White Plains, New York, on a special project at a well-known hospital. Of course, I accepted, not knowing everything it would bring with it. It just felt right. Have you ever had an opportunity come your way when everything in you tells you to go with it, even if you don't understand your *yes* in the moment you're making that decision? Even though everything around you seems like it's caving in on you. Your gut is confirming that you made the right choice, and all the green lights are flashing in your direction.

I call it the "check factor," meaning every box is checked and it's good to go. Sometimes not having a clear path but only blind faith can be enough to change your life (and become a bestselling author!) and cause you to hear yes far more often than no on your journey in an unexpected way. It won't be something you can explain; things you can explain are of this world, and things you cannot explain are from another world. Tap into that world and let your intuition guide you. It's a great place to be in, so don't be afraid to go with it—you might just enjoy the journey without knowing the results all at one time.

We humans love to have everything figured out before we take the leap of faith, but as we know, it doesn't play out like that. There is always the fear of the unknown. I believe everyone innately has intuition, but you must develop it to become stronger. It's just like muscles: if you don't build them, you will never see the benefits of a toned body. You will just be carrying around flesh and not feeling or experiencing your best life.

You never know what's around the corner when you decide to divorce fear. This fear-mate does nothing but take from your life—it never adds. So, before you get into this book, rid yourself of fear. Take a breath and enjoy the flight.

GOOD OLD PAPERWORK AND NON-COVERED EXPENSES

After my yes moment, I still had paperwork and those demanding onboarding requirements, which sometimes leave you exhausted and frustrated if not done in a timely manner. What was great about this assignment was that I had time to get it done; it was not a yes today and running the next day to meet all requirements. After everything was done, I was given the green light to begin work. Being a contractor has its advantages and disadvantages as to everything, but you make the best of it. One of the advantages most contractors have is that most expenses are either paid in full or covered by the employer.

In my case, my flight and expenses were paid by the company—which was a good thing because I had no money for any of it at the time, and that made it a little more difficult to navigate. I am a very private person; you would not know what is going on with me or my family if I didn't choose to tell you. I am a firm believer that family business is family business and not to be shared outside of the household. In the event that outside help is needed, hopefully you will be able to find one person you will feel comfortable bearing your soul to.

It was the season of life when I was in the middle of business transactions that were not coming as fast as I thought they should. I could not have moved the needle any faster if I wanted to, which caused anxiety and stress that not even ashwagandha could combat. For those who may not know about this herb, it has powerful medicinal therapeutic proprieties that help you in stressful times, and I urge you to go read about it and experience its wonders. Those of you who know about this herb can attest to how great it works with the body, especially if you are also on a plant-based diet—the wonderful feeling of ease in the body and mind. I have used ashwagandha when my body was full of toxins and processed foods, and I can attest that it doesn't work the same way as it does when your body is full of nutrients—you may get only half the benefits, if you're lucky.

I am a firm believer in having multiple streams of income, but most importantly, multiple streams of skills. When one skill is not needed, you can use another skill to make up for the lack. And that's what I did.

PREPARING TO TRAVEL

My assignment was starting in two weeks, enough time to get some chores done around the house and get things ready to travel. I had traveled over the last ten years, and one thing I loved about this assignment was the Monday–Thursday schedule. Being home on Fridays gave me a day to take care of personal appointments, something a "normal" schedule wouldn't enable you to do on a regular basis.

The day before my flight, for some reason I found myself running around doing more than I planned. Anyone who travels for work knows this is not the greatest strategy because you are bound to forget something. I made it through and got home at a decent hour to get my things packed and ready for the next day—but yes, I did forget an item or two.

SUNDAY MORNING

It was Sunday morning, time to get to the airport. When I woke up, I was somewhat not looking forward to traveling again, but I *was* counting my blessings that I was able to go on this assignment and make thousands of dollars in a matter of weeks. I could make as much money in a month as most people would in six months. Now that's skill-making!

After getting dressed and having something to eat, I called for an Uber. All the while, I was looking at my bank account and saying to myself and God, "Please don't let me run out of money for the next three weeks until I get paid." Yes, three weeks. I just happened to start on the pay week. As many of you know, if you start the pay week, you have an extra week to wait for your first paycheck, and for those who have started a job with little or no money, those three weeks can seem like a year. Even though my expenses were paid when it came to the hotel and flight, I was still responsible for the reimbursable miscellaneous items up front, and they would pay me on the back end. So I was on what is called a wing and a prayer for the entire three weeks. It was truly a faith walk. I did not reach out to my family or anyone.

To my surprise, this assignment would turn out to be a blessing in disguise. Sometimes in life we don't know where our journey will take us; we just need to be open to opportunities, and when you have that gut feeling, go with it—there is a bigger purpose than you can imagine.

My Uber driver was very friendly and made my ride to the airport enjoyable. After I was dropped off, I headed inside, thinking, *here we go again back in those friendly skies.* That's only if you like flying! If not, there is nothing friendly about the skies. Truth be told, I don't think most people like to fly. It's just a quick mode of transportation, and so we do it out of convenience. Some places you will never reach unless you fly, so if you choose not to take the occasional flight or two, you are cheating yourself out of enjoying this great planet we live on. I'm not saying travel the world but go to a couple of places on your bucket list before transitioning from this life.

THE AIRPORT

I got my ticket and headed to check in my bag, all the while thinking, *Another payment … this is one day I really could use that Sky Priority membership.* I just knew they were going to charge me for my bag because I didn't have the status I had before Covid.

I went up to the counter and put my luggage on the scale. It was heavier than I thought, and though I was only charged thirty dollars, at the time it felt like the agent was putting three times that amount on my card. (Readers who have been in this situation can attest to feeling overwhelmed when you have no control of the situation because of money.) Then I headed to TSA to be screened.

Anyone who has traveled to Hartsfield International knows it can be a nightmare, especially on Sundays and Mondays, though weekday travel is not as busy. To my surprise, I got TSA PreCheck, which gave me an advantage in that I didn't have to take my shoes off, along with a few perks more than regular check-in, and as we all know that helps, especially on busy days and tight flights.

When I was finally done with pre-check, I headed to the gate. At this point, I wasn't noticing anything different about myself. It seemed like the good old days. Little did I know that I would have a wake-up call in the weeks to come.

I reached the gate and had a little time until boarding. The first thing most frequent flyers do is go to the restroom, especially if the flight is more than a couple of hours long, so you don't have to get up and move around the plane. The plane I was flying on seated only about a hundred people, and it was not only a small plane but a tight one, the kind that you cannot put a roller bag on. You have to leave it on the jet bridge to go under the plane. An experienced avid flyer is like a person who knows cars, which ones to buy or not to buy. It's just another mode of transportation, and we should know what we are flying in and not just be a person that flies in the friendly skies.

I always try to get a window seat close to the front because I don't like the noise and cold at the back of the plane. I'm a flyer who doesn't like to talk to anyone. I say hello and then take my seat. I put my shades on if the person I will be sitting next to is already seated. Once I put my seat belt on, my shades are on, and my head is turned to the window. And honestly, I don't wake up until the flight lands, a flight attendant wakes me, or the pilot announces arrival.

Some of my closet friends will sometimes ask me, "How do you sleep when you're flying?" I answer, "I love it because God forbid anything happens, I will be in heaven before you can blink your eye if it does." I am not afraid of death. There is a time to be born and a time to die. Let's face it, we all must leave this planet one day only to transition to another. We must remember—not in fear, but to live the life we were created to live—that we are spiritual beings having a human experience. Those who are connected to Mother Nature and who eat the way we were designed to are set up for a more peaceful and serene life.

But before I got to this point, I didn't know what peaceful or serene even looked like. I was always anxious and nervous about everything and anything, running around in a state of chaos and confusion and not able to apply wisdom in the areas of my life that needed it the most. These emotions were bottled up inside me and were somewhat unexplainable to anyone in my circle of influence. Before committing to a plant-based diet, I didn't know I would ever feel this kind of freedom. As I will attest in this book, there is no other way to live an abundant life. We were created to live clean and healthy lives, not lives filled with processed and junk foods, but the way God intended from the beginning of time.

JUST LANDED

When I landed in White Plains and walked off the jet bridge, I was very surprised at such a small airport in New York. I thought the airport would be somewhat the size of LaGuardia. Looking around, I saw there was only one stop to pick up your luggage. That was a good thing for me now, because I really wasn't in the mood to be running around a big airport in twenty-degree weather. My frame of mind was partially because I was not eating live foods, as I would learn in the weeks to come.

I was exercising, but that is only about 20 percent of living a full and healthy life. If you're eating habits are not good, exercise really won't matter—you are not going to be able to think or hear clearly, let alone process any information or make good decisions. Your life will be foggy, and your decision-making will be the same because you are not feeding the brain and body what it takes to think clearly and function at an optimal level. I know, because today I am in a better place. The only way to find out is to make the decision; for me, the wake-up call came sooner rather than later.

I picked up my car and headed to the hotel. This part of New York was different from what I expected, having lived in New Jersey for about twelve years. It was very suburbia, somewhat country, compared to what I was used to. Even though I had gone to New York a lot when I was living in New Jersey, I never visited White Plains. It was always the city, mostly Manhattan and Brooklyn.

As I was driving down the highway, it was refreshing to be in a different environment. I was not on a clear path yet, but I still had a little sanity to enjoy the beauty of nature, although it was a cold and rainy night in New York.

I love nature, so however it comes, I roll with it. We are not always going to have sunny days in life. I believe that weather shows us how to be adaptable in life and how to move according to what the day brings. I am pretty sure we have heard the song "Fairweather Friend"—a fair-weather friend being one who is only going to be around when it's sunny. (I'm sure most of us can attest to this phenomenon.) I also believe that nature teaches us not only how to eat but also how to thrive and survive through whatever the circumstances are at the time.

Those who are not already plant-based may have been drawn in by the title of this book because you are considering a plant-based lifestyle. If you are plant-based already, you may be curious about whether my journey was like yours. (Either way, thank you for investing in me.) The thing to know is that you can change your way of eating and start seeing result in less than a week. It doesn't take a long time, nor is it complicated. To be honest, is it quite the opposite. It's a simple lifestyle that brings so much joy and alleviates the back-and-forth indecisiveness that causes a person to be in a state of confusion. I encourage you to experience the benefits of living a plant-based lifestyle immediately.

Only when you start eating "live" will you have true abundance, the abundance that gives you peace and tranquility to navigate this life. Friends and family may try to steer you from going down this path according to their own rationale or because they haven't experienced this lifestyle and have no desire to do so. My advice to you is to go with your gut and follow your mind.

Some might even argue that living a plant-based lifestyle is too expensive. I beg to differ. I say it's the opposite, because investing in your health can keep you from going down the path of sickness and disease. No matter how much money you earn, it will not keep you from having health issues if you are not putting the right things in your body. We all have seen very wealthy people who did not take care of their bodies. I'm sure when they get an unfavorable diagnosis, they probably say to themselves, *well, I have enough money to get me out of this situation*, but that's not always the case. I find that the wealthiest people in truth are those who may not have much when it comes to material possessions, but who eat healthily, make good decisions, and have a better quality of life.

The first thing admit is, I should have made different lifestyle choices, especially in eating. Start now making healthy lifestyle choices if you're not already doing so. For those who have no life-threatening conditions, congratulations. For those readers who may be may be dealing with a diagnosis, you can help turn it around by making better lifestyle choices. I believe there is hope for anyone who is alive, even if that means just starting today—tomorrow is not promised to anyone.

HOTEL ARRIVAL

I arrived at the hotel, thinking, *I hope the incidental for the entire stay is only twenty-five dollars*, and lo and behold, it was twenty-two dollars a night. I did not take this news well, knowing I had to pay out of pocket up front and then be reimbursed later.

Looking down at both cards in my wallet, I struggled to pick the right one for the front desk person to swipe, the one with the most money left on it. I reluctantly gave the clerk my card of choice, and he proceeded to charge my card *eighty-eight dollars* for the entire week's stay. I'm thinking, *please, Lord, no more incidentals this week—I still have food to buy.*

At this time, I was still eating processed and junk food. As we know, you can always find a deal at your local grocery store or fast-food restaurant. Unbeknownst to me, I was not making my situation better. My poor lifestyle choices were making it worse. Remember, that wake-up call was still weeks to come. You may be on the right path, but just don't know it until the light-bulb moment when you discover it.

After getting checked in, I headed to my room and settled in. I started searching for restaurants in the app to see what I could find that wasn't expensive. Lo and behold, I came across a few plant-based restaurants.

Although I had not begun a plant-based lifestyle yet, I always ate fruits and vegetables when they were available, along with processed and junk food—what a combination, as I look back. So it was always in my heart to go plant-based; I just never made the decision to do it until my wake-up moment came. Everyone I knew always said to me, "You eat so healthily," and it's true that I loved fruits and vegetables. And I thought I didn't have any life-threatening health issues. But there was one health issue, which we will discuss later in the book, that most people look at as not life-threatening but as normal—if you're not on medication for it, it must not be life-threatening.

I found a restaurant to order from that seemed perfect. I ordered a black bean burger with avocado, a strawberry shake (it was with almond or oat milk but a little high in calories), and to top it off, fried sweet potatoes, not baked. My old way of thinking was, *It's sweet potatoes, and they are healthy for you*. I got hooked on this one restaurant and ordered a different meal daily with different sides. This place was not cheap, but there were promotions that brought down the price enough that I was able to afford it. It really was the pleasure of the assignment, since a new job for the first couple of weeks is not really work but onboarding, which can sometimes be stressful, so therefore you need a healthy outlet.

I deluded myself into thinking that what I had to eat all week was good. I ate good food, yet I was fooling myself because I wasn't really eating healthily. Society wants you to think you can do just a little and still get a lot, but that's far from the truth. Living a plant-based lifestyle requires you to give up a lot at first and reap the benefits later. This advice may not make any sense until you make the change, but I'm confident that those who are already living a plant-based lifestyle can attest that you get what you put in.

You have a chance today to change. My light-bulb moment hadn't come yet. I was still eating what I wanted, traveling every week, and doing the things people do when travelling for work. I continued to go about week after week, living in the dark. There was no natural light, but I am a testament to the spiritual life being stronger than the dark. So in reading this book, let your light come on. The day your light comes on, you will be able to walk down a path that will bring you so much abundance, clarity, freedom, knowledge, and joy.

But this lifestyle is not something that can just be preached. You must live it to the fullest. If you don't, your actions, body, decision-making, and so many other aspects of your life will be lacking. It's like being born again. You are washed of the pollutants from the world's lifestyle of eating. You had chosen to participate in eating fast and processed foods, and if your choice is to go another direction, what I call a clear and narrow path, don't be surprised if only a few follow. It's not a path that seems rewarding in the moment, but it yields good fruit. It can feel like a boring path to be on at times if most people we know are making a different lifestyle choice that is contrary to how we were designed to live. I don't say this to condemn anyone; contrary to popular belief, the purpose of this eating lifestyle is not to condemn others. It's freeing. It frees the way we think from what society has said.

Let's discuss food addiction. We know that processed food and sugar are like drugs; they keep you bound and hooked until you decide to get to get free. It's not an easy decision. Society is your worst enemy, but you are your first enemy. You are saying to yourself, "I don't deserve to live a good and fruitful life—my body doesn't deserve it." But what if I told you your body deserves it, and more?

I can tell you that, but you are the only one who can make the change. No matter how many books you read or how many videos you watch on social media, the only person who can change your lifestyle of eating is *you*. I'm not telling you to become fully plant-based all at once, as I did. But I am telling you to decide to live a healthier life going forward and to the enjoy the fruits of it.

8

FROM HPN TO ATL

As I mentioned in earlier chapters, I was just going through the motions until I started traveling and eating, including the good stuff. I can remember my wake-up call so well. It was a holiday week, with cancellations and everything that can be encountered during this time, and the airport was crowded. I sat down with my laptop and belongings next to a passenger who was very friendly, and we began to talk. Our flight was delayed, and we enjoyed our conversation and waited patiently for our arrival. Finally, we were told on the intercom that our plane had arrived—to our amazement, since this airport shuts down when the weather is not conducive for flying. Little did I know that my journey to a plant-based lifestyle was also beginning.

The other traveler and I got up and proceeded to the gate. We mentioned to each other that we wished we were sitting together on the plane. We asked the gate attendant to check for other available seating, but because this flight was overbooked, no arrangements could be made. We said our goodbyes and went our separate ways prior to boarding.

As I proceeded down the aisle, I had to turn somewhat to the side. At the time, I thought, *oh, it's just these bags in my hand, and that's why I can't get through the aisle.* This was my only thinking, because I was still operating in darkness.

When I reached my seat, the person I was assigned to sit next to was already seated. He got up and let me in. It was a struggle getting into my seat—not only to sit down but to fasten my seat belt. And that's when the light bulb came on. I could not believe that I was seating myself on a plane and could hardly buckle my seat belt. But to my surprise, the person next to me didn't seem to notice. He didn't need to; I did. I was in a state of shock to recognize that I had let myself get to a point where *I could not fasten my seat belt.*

I finally got my seat belt buckled, but I felt such weight on me—what I would more accurately call bondage. I was truly bound by a lifestyle of poor eating. I said to myself, *You are going to have to do something about this.* My income depended on traveling, and I had to do everything in my power to maintain it. I had business transactions that had not come through yet, but that was doing me no good now but keeping hope alive. *This is serious,* I continued to say to myself, *and you do not want to be embarrassed by getting on a flight some day and not being able to buckle your seat belt.* From my experience, most people are not warm and friendly on planes.

It was a humbling moment for me. I remembered times when someone who was overweight had sat next to me like that, how it was such a struggle for them to buckle their seat belt and get comfortable—well, as comfortable as anyone can be on a plane. I have even seen the person pretend they are strapped in, only to put themselves in danger if an emergency happens. All the while, they are miserable and cannot wait for the plane to land. The reason I can say that is because I said it myself on that rainy night flying from HPN to Hartsfield.

PATRICIA A. MORGAN

ANOTHER ONE BITES THE DUST

I couldn't go another day feeling that way. I was tired all the time, going back and forth to my doctor's office. When you're going through darkness, no one understands it. Doctors want to medicate the symptoms because they don't know how to treat what they cannot see. It left me frustrated to leave the office the same way I came. The only thing my doctor knew to do was to prescribe medications based on what I was trying to explain. She didn't perform blood work because she was used to me coming into the office every couple of months saying the same old thing over and over.

"What seems to be the problem?" she would ask.

My answers were always the same: "I don't feel well," "I'm tired," and so on.

She would go on to prescribe this and that, saying we would "see if it takes care of the symptoms you are experiencing."

But I would not pick up my prescriptions at the pharmacy. I was not a walking pharmacy. I would not accept that. I knew I could do better, but at the time I did not know the route to take. I was so frustrated that I began to think there was no hope. I felt miserable. I was not buying the commonplace notion that "these things happen when you get to a certain age." It was much more than that. I wasn't straight out of high school, but I hadn't graduated from college yet either, if you catch my drift.

The light was shining, but I didn't know it yet. During my most recent visit to the doctor's office, I told her I felt that I needed to change my eating habits. "You need to have thirty grams of protein a day," she advised me.

"I don't like eating that much meat a day," I said. I preferred fruits and vegetables, nuts and seeds, and grains.

"That's not going to work," she insisted. "You need more than that to sustain a healthy lifestyle. If you are not willing to eat chicken and beef, then have salmon. No meat is not an option." Then she repeated, "You must have at least thirty grams of protein daily."

Of course, I looked at her with my daddy's eyes and nodded.

I felt like I was fighting a losing battle. It was the same thing over and over every time I would go for my visit. I made up my mind not to go back there and not to take what she recommended. I decided to find another doctor who would be more understanding and not try to put me on all sorts of meds. It was time to make a change.

THE ART OF STILLNESS

The truth, I would learn later, was that it wasn't up to her to make me feel good. It was up to me. But because I was in the dark, I didn't really know how to do that. I was on to something, though I wasn't yet fully aware of it, when I expressed to her what I thought I should be eating. It just goes to show that your intuition or gut, whatever you want to call it, can lead you in the right direction, if you just slow down, breathe, and listen. There is magic in stillness.

As a society we have it twisted. We think running around all the time, doing all sorts of things, is productive. It's the opposite: it's counterproductive. You have to decide to make stillness in your life—not quietness, and there is a difference. You might be told to be quiet; to be still is your decision. You hold the power to decide to be still in a way that will add to the abundance of life.

I'm not saying this choice will be easy, but I guarantee you that everyone who lives this way will attest to having a balanced life. It's not a lifestyle about holding yourself to certain rules and regulations. It's not a life that restricts you or makes you feel like you are missing out on something. It is a spiritual practice, a way of preserving the temple.

But you are not making the decision solely for you. You are taking care of the planet at the same time. I believe that is what we were called to the earth to do, to till the ground and live an abundant life, not just live to obtain and hoard material possessions. Material possessions do not do a body good; they give the mind a quick dose of dopamine only to let it go back to its normal way of thinking in days.

If people really look at what material things are costing them when they do not live a balanced life, they would be better able to find ways to change and to live a life of abundance rather than stress. Materialism is not what I would call a fulfilling life. It's a life that's downright false: it gives people false expectations, it lures the soul, and it causes confusion, jealousy, hoarding, pride, and all manner of evil.

KEEP IT 3

My son has a brand called Keep It 3, which deals with first the spiritual, then with health, and last wealth. I love the concept because it shows the balance and order of the three. I love the fact that his mind was open enough to receive this download and to give to the world a picture of what a balanced life looks like.

If we are to live this kind of life, we must lay down every false way— in a nutshell, get rid of it! Start living an authentic life, a life that's pleasing to yourself and others. And yes, yourself first: unless you take care of yourself, you will not have the capacity to take care of others. I am speaking from experience. You will not be able to focus on the most important thing that's right in front of you; in other words, your focus will be off.

This is one of the keys to living a plant-based lifestyle, a life that empowers others, makes them feel appreciated and loved, and makes you feel good when you take care of your temple, wealthy in more than just material things. The greatest gift you can give to yourself and others is to maintain a healthy lifestyle. I call it the "aphrodisiac of the planet"! It doesn't feel or get any better than this.

FLIPPING THE SWITCH

I flipped the switch, and life began to change. It started first in the mind. What an eye-opener! The next day, after landing home, I changed immediately. It was instant, just as when you flip the switch, and the light comes on. That's how it was for me, anyway. I acted immediately, and I did not hesitate. It was necessary; I would say downright urgent.

Sometimes we can face life-changing decisions that will change the trajectory of our lives for good or bad. It all depends on the individual and how they look at the situation. For example, two people can face the same situation and have totally different outcomes. It comes down to the person's choice. No two people will have the same result.

I try not to approach a situation by saying, "It's supposed to happen this way," or by asking, "Will it ever happen that way?" Individuals have their own God-given right to think and do. We are all human beings with free will, and that will never change as long as we exist on this planet. Whether you use your free will for the good of yourself or others, or do the opposite, it's a choice.

I hope this chapter will imbue you with the desire to make whatever choices are necessary to get the results you're looking for.

FROM THE PLANE
TO THE PLANET

Now we get down to why this book was written. This book grew from a transformative event. I've talked about seating myself on the plane and how uncomfortable and difficult it was for me to buckle my seat belt. That was the eye-opener for me to make a swift decision to lose weight and cut all the junk from my life. This junk was not benefiting me spiritually or naturally, and it was affecting me mentally as well.

Usually I'm asleep before the plane takes off. This trip was different. I could not get comfortable. Sure, there was a young child kicking the back of my seat the entire trip, but that was not the issue. My body was telling me it was time to make a change. Not in words, of course, but in my tossing and turning the whole trip home. For the next two hours, I thought about the change that needed to take place. It was high time I did something.

I went back to that last conversation with my doctor about eating habits. If I did not change my eating habits, I knew I was going to have some serious health issues down the road. I could not afford that, not with all the great things that were happening for me at the time and that lay in the days ahead. I could not afford to be physically unable to sit in the seat of an airplane or be embarrassed when traveling. My livelihood was at stake, and excuses were out the window. This was a live-or-die situation.

We don't often see being overweight as a diagnosis, but it is. We see weight as part of the person, but it's deeper than the eye. It's a diagnosis because it affects the body's organs. It's one of the diagnoses that brings on other problems for us to deal with—for instance, it's a culprit in diseases that involve inflammation.

But my doctor never told me being overweight was a diagnosis. I found out through my own research. My doctor always told me to work on getting my weight and BMI down in order to live a more productive life, but she failed to mention this diagnosis labeled "overweight." In my experience, there have been small conversations *around* rather than *on* this topic.

Finding out that being overweight was an actual diagnosis was yet another eye-opener. I'm glad I was able to diagnose myself. Some of you may be dealing with other diagnoses, but when it comes down to it, many if not all could be reversed by sticking to a cleaner way of living.

14

BACK HOME

My flight arrived back at Hartsfield international airport. It was a somewhat short flight, and I had used the restroom before boarding, but I needed to go to the restroom after I got off the jet bridge. Going through the airport was somewhat challenging. As I walked, all the while I kept saying to myself that tomorrow would be the start of a new day. After I went to the restroom and got my luggage, I called an Uber.

After arriving home, I found that I had received the detox and colon cleanse I had ordered before leaving. I had told myself I needed a cleanse. I thought a cleanse would help me feel better, but if your eating is not on point, as mine was not at the time, a cleanse is not going to help much. You will need to change your eating habits for a cleanse to be fully effective.

Since I had already made up my mind to go cold turkey plant-based the next day, getting the cleanse was good timing. Before I had even taken the trip and had my realization, I had been reading a great plant-based lifestyle book—again I was being guided—so I knew exactly what I was going to buy at the supermarket.

The next morning, I woke up bright and early, got dressed, and headed out to the store. I had my list, and I was so excited to have a plan in place to buy what I needed to get started, thanks to a great book and the community I had joined as part of my book purchase and detox cleanse. I felt so good shopping; for the first time, I was not all over the place, trying to decide between the junk and the good food available for me to choose from.

I was also clear with my thoughts because I had not eaten yet. I didn't have anything in my house that went along with my new lifestyle. I believe intermittent fasting works because when you fast, your mind is clear and sharp, and so you make very precise decisions. What was great about this shopping trip was that I stayed mostly on the outskirts of the supermarket, expecting to get my spring water, nuts, seeds, and oils. I had never been one to go shopping and enjoy it, but I enjoyed shopping for the first time.

After browsing the areas and making sure everything on my list was obtainable, I began shopping in earnest. Looking at the variety of vegetables and fruits, and the beauty of their colors and what they represented, I was fascinated. I had never really *looked* at fruits and vegetables that way before. I had been eating them my whole life but had not truly appreciated these God-given foods. I picked up every item one by one, inspecting everything I picked up. I felt a shift happening as I set my intentions on getting healthy.

I thought losing weight was my priority, but I would find out in the weeks to come that it really wasn't. At the core, it's about getting healthy. Once I started eating right, with no effort I began to shed the weight. What I experienced as weight loss is a by-product of what really happens: you begin to change from the inside out. Your thoughts, decisions, conversations, work, sleep—all begin to be much clearer. I was able to finish a book in a matter of days when in the past it probably would have taken me months.

I was so excited about the decision I had made. I began putting my personal and professional goals together, and they finally made sense to the point where I could see myself achieving them. This comes from self-knowledge. You can be gifted, and as we all know, writing is one of the gifts given to mankind, but you will not be able to execute any of your goals if your mind and spirit are not in harmony. Not accomplishing your goals can only lead to frustration, burn out, and sometimes giving up, if you're not careful. I am truly thankful this was not my ending, though it is for some. I kept moving and getting things accomplished. To my amazement, I was checking off my list of things that I had completed daily. Just to name a few, I joined a wonderful community which we called "the tribe," and my clothes were so loose I had to go shopping.

I felt good about that last one, because one of my goals was to go out of the country for vacation and to shed some weight before the spring. I made it happen and was able to visit the country of Belize. I began to shed everything around me that did not serve my highest purpose according to the plan I had put in place. I removed everything—including but not limited to people, places, and things—and for the first time, to my surprise, there was no condemnation or guilt about it.

Another benefit of the plant-based lifestyle was that I became very patient in my actions, which was not normal for me. We have all heard the word "proactive," but being proactive can be a good thing or a bad thing. For example,

I was scheduled to head out for work the following week. Usually, I would get my itinerary email with flight, hotel, and rental per my request in advance. But after having submitted it more than four days before I was supposed to leave, to my surprise, I had not received it by the day before. The old me would have panicked; I would have called my company asking where my next week's itinerary was: "The client is expecting me to be on site!" This time, I did not panic, nor did I call or have any anxiety about the situation. I had done what was required. *If I am not on site for this client next week, it's no fault of my own*, I told myself.

I waited until five o'clock Friday and never received my email with the details for the next week's travel. Again, I did not call or panic at all. Ordinarily, I would have called them by noon to ask where my itinerary is, and if I didn't get an answer, I would email—I would get this resolved, come hell or high water. But because I was in a different space spiritually, mentally, and physically, I neither called nor emailed. I was not going to run down people to get them to do their job, and I surely was not going to pay out of pocket and get reimbursed for the trip, though by this time I could afford to pay for my expenses. I planned to contact the client by email to let them know what happened and that I was still open to working remotely.

The day came, and I did just as I told myself I would do. I sent an email letting the client know what had happened and requested a Zoom meeting to discuss the project. They really didn't have a choice but to be OK with it. I knew the software I was training their providers on, and they needed me at the time. Either way, I was not anxious about the situation, whichever way it would turn out.

To be honest, I did not mind not receiving my travel documents by email. I had gotten used to working remotely for a while with permission of the client, and I really wasn't looking forward to going back to traveling. As we all know, Covid-19 dramatically increased the number of people able to work remotely, and this experience has made remote work more acceptable than in the past. It's no longer outside the norm to work from home—if anything, it has become the norm with some kinds of work. I personally don't ever think we will go back to the old way of doing things. We are now in what I consider a new and evolving way to live.

GETTING BACK ON THE PLANE

The following week I was about to head back to New York, anticipating the joy and excitement I would feel once I got back on a plane. I was excited to be flying again. I don't think I got much sleep the night before. I couldn't wait to see how I felt getting on the plane and how comfortable I would be sitting after losing so much weight. It wasn't about the weight; it was about how I felt, but in this case my weight was the determining factor in how I would feel once I got back on a plane and took my seat.

The next morning finally came. I got up in a great mood. Plant-based living will give you a great temperament, if you don't have one already. I got dressed and called for my Uber. It was like the driver just couldn't come fast enough. I was only ten minutes from the airport, but to me it felt like an hour.

When I dashed through the airport this time, I was not breathing hard or feeling weighed down. I got my ticket, took my bags to the check-in counter (well able to pay for it all by now), and went through TSA and to my assigned gate, skipping all the way in anticipation. To my chagrin, the flight was delayed. I shook my head and said to myself, *Why today? Any other day it would be on time.* Not only was my flight delayed, it had to be checked for unexpected maintenance.

This surely can't be happening to me, I thought, *the day I'm back in the air as a new person with a new wardrobe and hair.* (Another gem: a plant-based lifestyle does wonders for hair.) I tried to wait patiently; honestly, I didn't have a choice. After about an hour, the gate agent finally made an announcement that we would be taking another plane because ours could not be fixed in time. We were instructed to grab our bags and head to Gate D21. I stood up with no hesitation. I was in great shape now and at this point was ready to get on any plane that was flying that day.

I started walking fast across the airport, passing by all the restaurants full of cakes, cookies, pies, and processed foods. I could count on my hands the number of plant-based eating places, maybe two out of ten. One day I hope to see airports offer a better selection of every form of lifestyle eating. It's high time people became more educated about the different lifestyles and not be limited to one or two ways of eating. We're doing somewhat better but have a long way to go. Let's put forth the effort as plant-based eaters to see more options. We are a mighty and growing community, so let's keep up the good work.

When I finally arrived at the new gate, the agent announced they were cleaning the plane and we would be boarding in about twenty minutes. I took that time to use the restroom so I wouldn't have to in the air. I like to sleep the entire trip, regardless of the length of the flight; I only wake up when the plane is about to land. Now that's cruising the friendly skies!

The gate agent finally announced that we were boarding. I had been waiting for this day for quite a while. Those of us who fly know the rules: you must wait your turn. But I stood up to get in line with those flying first class, children, and special needs passengers. I wanted to get on the plane as fast as possible. So when the gate agent finally called my section, there was no need for me to get in line—I was already up and waiting. As I headed down the jet bridge, I'm more leaping than walking. There were other people waiting to get on the plane, but there was not a long a wait.

Once on the plane, as a frequent flyer I knew pretty much where I would be sitting based on my seat number. I walked through first class and got about a third of the way down the aisle when I realized, *You did not tap one person on the left or right.* I continued to my seat. *You didn't touch anyone.* I smiled and put my things in the overhead with no struggle.

There was no one in the seat next to mine yet, so I proceeded to take my seat. I felt just as I imagined I would: amazed at how effortlessly my seat belt went on and how there was room left in the seat next to me, even though this was not a big plane and the space was small. I was smiling to myself at the person I had become inside and out. I had been able to experience my transformation. It was a big change compared to what I experienced the last time I was flying!

My flight was wonderful. I think even the person who sat beside me was more comfortable. The flight was not turbulent but smooth all the way—a good thing when you're 33,000 feet in the air, though for those who don't like flying at all, this may be relative. No change of weight will cause me not to sleep, though the quality is sure to be affected. Staying awake is not an option for me, as I have trained my body to sleep when it's in the air, just as we train our bodies to do anything. We are the masters of our temple; we can control or not control what we choose to put in our bodies. Today I can say I am happy that I control my body, and it does not control me. I feel good knowing I am the master of my destiny, the captain of my ship.

Finally, the announcement came on: "We are now beginning our descent into HPN." I awoke from my slumber to get prepared for landing. Upon landing, my experience getting off the plane was as satisfying as getting on. I got my own luggage, and I didn't encounter any issues getting through the aisle. But I wasn't as excited about getting off the plane as I was getting on. I wanted to linger and luxuriate in my feeling of success. I had accomplished a major goal, and it was paying off more richly than I could have imagined. I said goodbye to the crew a little sadly, and headed to get my bags and rental car.

After arriving at the hotel, I did not order any food other than what I had become accustomed to. There is something about going plant-based: not only do your taste buds change, your appetite does as well. The next morning, I got dressed for work and headed out the door. The breakfast at the hotel I stay at usually includes some type of fruit, surrounded by junk and processed foods. I was able to pick the good out of the bad. I had some blueberries and melon and hot chamomile tea to start my day.

My client was a hospital. As I walked through the door, my colleagues were out front instead of downstairs where they usually are in the morning. They all gave me with such a stare. I knew what it was. I didn't say anything, but all the while I'm laughing inside. Everyone was looking, but no one said what they were thinking. They just greeted me with how they had missed me and were glad I was back after such a long time.

"I'm glad to be back to be back," I responded.

16

TRAVELING HOME
FROM HPN TO ATL

The time for traveling home had arrived, and I headed to the airport. I wasn't as excited as I had been about the trip there. I didn't think a few days would make any difference in the experience flying back, but it did—not in getting into my seat but who was sitting next to me. My seatmate this time was a heavy person who had to use some of my seating space in addition to their own.

That would usually irritate me a little, but because I was on my life's path, it didn't. My temperament was great. I had no complaints about how I had to position my body. Usually I would feel like I was trying to get out the window so I wouldn't be touched.

Because of what I had achieved, I was able to be somewhat comfortable and to sleep the whole way. My experience was great from the plane to the planet!

FLYING ACROSS THE WORLD

I am so happy to say that flying has become a pleasure for me and is no longer a dread. In the past year, I've been able to take vacations to places that were very quiet and peaceful, with plenty of sunshine and an array of great foods from the earth.

I have also written several other books this year to empower those who live on this planet. I look forward to continuing this successful journey and meeting with various plant-based communities and like-minded people all over the world. Always remember: *The minority is the majority.*

MY PLANT-BASED JOURNEY

My journey has been sweet. Because my mind was made up and I knew what I needed to do to take my life to abundance and prosperity, I would not say that it has been challenging. But I have learned a lot on my journey and still have more to learn in the days to come.

One of the most rewarding things for me was getting involved in my community and working with those who are interested in this way of living. I am convinced that this way of life is necessary and not merely a choice, if you want to sustain good health.

But there are many benefits to this daily lifestyle. Not only am I now the size I have always dreamt of being in terms of weight, but I began cooking healthier dishes for my family as well. I started traveling the world. My business endeavors went through the roof. Everything I did succeeded. Some of my future goals are to open my own herb shop and smoothie bar in my community to give back and pave the way for my family and future generations.

I'm not saying that a plant-based diet alone will do all this. There is work to be done on your part. There is action to all things, and eating cannot do everything. When you put it all together, it's magic. Wonderful things happen.

I hope that having read this book you will feel the same and make the change, or continue on your own plant-based journey with a stronger sense of purpose and community if you have already made the choice. The key is to just get started no matter where you are in life. Make the decision to make it happen.

I don't believe you purchased this book by accident. Get rid of all doubt and fear. These feelings only paralyze your life and stop you from achieving greatness. Walk out the greatness you were created for. Commit to coming in tune with your highest and best self.

I pray that you are blessed and empowered, and I am eternally grateful that you purchased my book. May you receive this love extended back to you. May whatever road you travel be peaceful and bright, and may all your dreams and desires come to fruition. May you never give up no matter what, knowing you can and will accomplish all you set out to do.

If you are already plant-based, I pray that you remain on the path of abundance. If you are not but are exploring the possibilities, I pray that this book has brought an awareness of what lies beyond what you can see today.

Many blessings,

TRANSITIONING TO A PLANT-BASED LIFESTYLE

Here are seven steps you can take to transition to your new plant-based lifestyle.

1. **Decide how you will make the transition**. Your transition will be based on your current lifestyle—for example, whether you're going from omnivore to plant-based, or from vegan to plant-based, or to go cold turkey and straight to a plant-based lifestyle. I did not want any substitutes. It was now or never for me. Most important is for you to be comfortable in your decision-making.

2. **Write it down.** Write down your vision, make it a plan, and run with it. Make it simple. There is no need to be all over the place with your decision to feed the body and keep the temple clean. There are certain foods you can eat, and certain foods that are not permitted.

3. **Join a community.** Find a community that values the same things you value, that will support you and give you great tools for this abundant life. That

includes but is not limited to restaurants that are plant-based, or meetings.

4. **Read books on the subject.** Find great books on plant-based eating and lifestyles. Books can help you with different recipes and a wealth of knowledge for your journey.

5. **Make a shopping list.** Especially in the beginning, take a list to the grocery store, whether in handwritten or digital form. Don't leave home without it, or you will end up picking up items that may not be plant-based or not be the type of foods you need to be eating.

6. **Cleanse and detox.** Find a good herbal cleansing detox online or at your local health food store.

7. **Get quality sleep and relaxation.** Give yourself quality time. Whether in the form of sleeping or just relaxing on the seashore, quality time does a body good.

SAMPLE SHOPPING LIST

Vegetables

kale

spinach

romaine or any lettuce
    but iceberg

cucumber

squash

bell peppers

mushrooms *(but not shitake)*

tomatoes, cherry and
    plum only

onions

olives

avocado

garbanzo beans, also
    known as chickpeas

okra

Fruits

blueberries

strawberries

blackberries

raspberries

pears

peaches

apples *(organic only)*

grapes

mangos *(my favorite!)*

bananas, small or medium

cantaloupe

limes

lemons

melons

raisins

dates

cherries

prunes

prickly pear

Grains

quinoa
wild rice
spelt
teff
kamut
fonio

Seasonings

basil
thyme
clove
pink Himalayan sea salt
cilantro
cayenne pepper
bay leaf
dill
turmeric
oregano

Nuts and seeds

almonds *(always presoak
    before consuming)*
pecans
Brazil nuts
flaxseed
hempseed
tahini

Sweeteners

pure agave (cactus) syrup
dates

Oils

avocado oil
sesame oil
hempseed oil
grapeseed oil
olive oil *(do not cook with)*
coconut oil *(do not cook with)*

Beverages

natural spring water★
coconut water straight from
    the coconut

★ *If you desire a little kick for
    your water, try infusers such
    as botanical hibiscus, mint,
    limes, lemons, strawberries,
    blueberries, or oranges*

Herbs and superfoods

chamomile
elderberry
turmeric root
gingerroot
sea moss
valerian
burdock *(one of my favorites!)*
chlorella
allspice
hemp
plant-based seed and nut
    milks, such as coconut
    milk, almond milk,
    flaxseed milk

MY FAVORITE AVOCADO DRESSING

Hats off to my community, who shared this recipe with me.

1 ripe avocado, peeled, pitted, and mashed
1/2 medium green pepper, finely chopped
2 tablespoons tahini
1 tablespoon pure agave nectar
1 pinch Himalayan sea salt
1 teaspoon coconut vinegar

Printed in the United States
by Baker & Taylor Publisher Services